Loving The Skin You're In

Loving The Skin You're In

YOUR ULTIMATE GUIDEBOOK
IN NOURISHING YOUR SKIN

• • •

Linda Irwin-Hurley

ISBN: 0692868437
ISBN 13: 9780692868430
Library of Congress Control Number: 2017910147
CreateSpace Independent Publishing Platform
North Charleston, South Carolina

Dedication

• • •

You are holding this book in your hand because of the encouragement I have received from all the people who believed in telling the story of skin and the importance of caring for it.

Acknowledgements

• • •

Black Card Books for the beautiful cover design.

Toni Steffen, Websites by Toni for her hard work in helping me get this book ready for print.

Rose Tring, AZ Media Maven LLC for her outstanding editing of the manuscript.

Lisa Henss, director of nutritional counseling and metabolic testing at Clairton Family Chiropractic for her guidance and editing of Chapter 6 on exercise and nutrition.

All the Nourish Your Skin Consultants and Customers who have given much needed encouragement, without them the book would never have reached completion.

Table of Contents

Disclaimer

• • •

THE AUTHOR OF THIS BOOK is not a licensed medical physician or dermatologist. The information provided in this book is solely the opinions of the author.

This book is not intended as a substitute for the medical advice of physicians. The reader should regularly consult a physician in matters relating to his/her health and particularly with respect to any symptoms that may require diagnosis or medical attention.

The content of this book is meant to be for informational purposes only and it is suggested that you do your own research before using any of the nutritional advice, products, or exercises mentioned.

Chapter 1

• • •

YOUR SKIN AND ITS FUNCTIONS

YOUR SKIN IS THE LARGEST and most amazing organ of your body, making it your most valuable asset. However, most of us take our skin for granted and do not give our skin the loving care it needs to perform at its peak potential.

Your skin covers your organs and protects your body from the outside elements, and it makes up about 16 percent of your body weight.

Give your skin the break it deserves because it serves as the protective barrier for your body.

THE THREE MAIN LAYERS OF SKIN

Layer one: The Epidermis
The epidermis is the outermost layer of the skin, consisting of five separate layers itself: *stratum basale*, the bottom or basal cell layer; *stratum spinosum*, squamous cell layer and thickest layer; the *stratum granulosum*, containing keratinocytes; the *stratum lucidum*, which is only on the palms of hands and the soles of our feet; and the *stratum corneum*, which is the outermost

and top layer, and made up of keratinocytes that shed about every two weeks.

The epidermis is the thinnest of the three major skin layers. Thickness varies from the thin covering on our eyelids to the thick layer on the palms of our hands and soles of our feet. The epidermis protects us from external irritation, prevents water loss and stops the entry of bacteria. Epidermal cells reproduce themselves on a 28-day cycle. The top dead skin cells are the body's natural process of exfoliation. With aging, our epidermis thins and the number of pigment-containing cells decreases. Aging skin looks thinner, paler, and translucent. We tend to get pigmented liver spots that appear in our sun-exposed areas.

Also, our connective tissue weakens with age and reduces the skin's strength and elasticity. We produce less of our natural oils, which can make it harder to keep our skin moist. The dead skin cells that we shed have little or no water, so older skin may feel dry and can easily chap, or in extreme cases, crack on the heels, elbows, and knees.

The epidermal layer also is the layer that determines skin color. The melanocytes (melanin or pigment) will determine whether you will have a fair or dark complexion.

Layer two: **The Dermis**

The dermis is the middle layer of skin. It is about ten times thicker that the epidermis. The dermis provides support and structure to skin. Within the dermal layer lives the connective tissue, containing collagen, which gives skin its firmness; elastic tissue, which gives skin its elasticity; and hyaluronic acid, which provides moisture to skin. Hair follicles, nerves, lymphatic vessels, oil glands, and sweat glands also reside in the dermal layer, which extends outward to the epidermal layer. The dermis is made up of 60 percent to 80 percent water and provides moisture to the epidermis.

Layer three: **The Subcutaneous tissue**

The subcutaneous tissue is the lower most layer of skin, and is made up mostly of fat. The subcutaneous tissue protects bones and muscles from injury, produces heat, and serves as a cushion for the body.

Skin acts as a heat exchanger to help our body maintain its temperature at around 98.6 degrees Fahrenheit by regulating the heat that is released through the skin. As body temperature rises, the capillary vessels beneath the skin's surface open and excess heat escapes through the skins' pores. If that is not enough to cool you, then your body will further reduce its temperature through perspiration via the sweat glands. If your body temperature is too cold then your capillaries will contract, which slows down the heat escaping from your body.

Our skin is our largest organ, and it provides protection, padding, warmth and cooling, and its nerves allow us to touch and feel. Pretty amazing, right?

WHAT IS MY SKIN TYPE?

Determining skin type is a leading question because some people confuse skin color with skin condition. Some skin may be darker, some may be lighter but the caring for any skin requires essential the same steps. Although, fairer skin may require additional sun protection than darker toned skin.

Skin color is generally divided into six shades:

1. Extremely fair with light eyes and hair – extremely prone to sunburn. People with red and pale blonde fall into this category, and must take every precaution when venturing into the sun.

2. Fair with medium dark hair and eyes – usually burns, sometimes tans. Brunettes, or dark blondes with brown eyes might fit this category, which must still be careful when in direct sun.

3. Medium, olive, or golden skin, medium dark hair, and dark eyes – may burn, usually tans. People with dark and darker skin tones may not have to worry as much about burning, but without protection the sun still is damaging to their skin.

4. Deeper olive skin with dark hair and eyes – rarely burns, always tans. Again, this skin tone typically doesn't burn, but that doesn't mean going outside without using property sunscreen.

5. Dark brown skin with dark hair and eyes – tans easily, rarely burns. Again, burning is not likely, but any skin that has no protection faces an increased risk of sun damage.

6. Black skin and hair, dark eyes – rarely burns. Just because there is little likelihood of burning, doesn't mean you can go without protection. All shades of skin must be protected while in direct sunlight, although darker skin won't require as much protection as lighter skin does.

Your skin color stays close to the same, especially if you use protection to avoid damaging your skin with tanning. However, the condition of your skin can change from day-to-day, or even within the same day depending on the weather, your health, and other variables.

There are different types of skin, and that is determined by the amount of sebum—an oily, waxy substance—that skin secretes and the amount of moisture each type of skin retains.

There are two main zones of the face:

1. T-Zone – Forehead and nose
2. U-Zone – The cheeks, jawline and chin.

The following are four different examples of variable skin conditions:

Normal Skin: The T-Zone secretes sebum at a moderate rate. The U-Zone has sufficient moisture.

Dry Skin: The T-Zone secretes sebum at a moderate rate. The U-Zone lacks moisture.

Oily Skin: The T-Zone creates excess sebum. The U-Zone has sufficient moisture.

Combination Skin: The T-Zone produces excess sebum. The U-Zone lacks moisture.

Depending on your complexion and your skin condition, you will need to take certain steps to preserve and care for your skin. Do you take the proper care of your skin? Remember, "the better we take care of our skin, the better it will take care of us." The following chapters will guide you on the best way to care for your beautiful skin.

Chapter 2

• • •

YOU AND YOUR SKIN

DURING A TYPICAL WEEK, MY business takes me to numerous independent and assisted living facilities. These are my favorite places to visit and one of the reasons I have chosen skin care as a means of helping humanity. The elderly residents are a wealth of information on subjects of the past and present. I have met many people who I would have guessed to maybe be in their 80s, with their quick minds and quick steps, only to find out they may be approaching their 100th birthdays. Conversing with them is like stepping into a history book. But when you ask the simple question, "Do you have dry skin," about 80 percent will tell you no. The simple answer, though, is that of course they do.

Unfortunately, this belief that their skin has plenty of moisture is not restricted to elderly people. In working many farmers' markets, I would ask the public the same question and I would get similar answers. Skin is the largest organ in our bodies, but it is taken for granted most often and frequently neglected. We bake it, we put chemicals on it, and we starve it.

Here are some general rules about caring for skin each day. All skin has a tendency toward dehydration. In extreme cases, dry skin lacks elasticity and can be extremely sensitive to the sun, wind, and cold temperatures. To help keep skin healthy, wash your face at least once a day with a rich, organic facial cleanser that has no sulfates, and warm water. Pat your skin dry and use a non-alcohol toner that will not dry out your skin. Follow with a crème-based moisturizer to hydrate your skin and keep it rejuvenated.

Pay special attention to fragile areas such as eyes and lip areas. These areas of your face are more sensitive and deserve special attention. The skin around the eyes is ten times finer than the skin on the rest of the face. It is important to start using an eye crème as early as your 20s. I suggest a rich emollient that will help prevent early eye crinkles, reduce the sag in the upper eye lid, and help with dark circles and puff on the skin directly below your eye. For the fine skin on your lips, find an organic lip balm that is compatible to your lips and don't hesitate to reapply to this particularly fragile area as often as necessary.

Use an organic exfoliation to wash with as a granular cosmetic preparation will assist in removing dead cells from the skin's surface. I recommend treatment once or twice a week. It must be effective, yet gentle and respectful of the tender skin of our faces.

Moisturizing is essential. The dermis (inner layer) is made up of 70 percent water and the epidermis (outer layer), 15 percent. To keep the skin moisturized, it is important to choose a daily moisturizing organic skin care product that will balance the level of water within the skin. I recommend using a product that contains hyaluronic acid and aloe vera.

Also, always use sunscreen and drink lots of water. The recommended water intake per day is half your body weight in ounces. (For example, if you weigh 140 pounds, you should drink at least 70 ounces of water per day.)

Pollution, smoke, stress etc. - all have harmful effects on the skin. Use organic skincare products to protect your skin against these daily stresses before leaving the house and cleanse your skin thoroughly when you come home in the evening.

Chapter 3

• • •

WHY ORGANICS?

WHY USE ORGANIC / NON-TOXIC PRODUCTS?

ONE OF MY MOST FREQUENTLY asked questions; "Why organics"?

Well, the first and foremost answer to that question is simple. Your skin is porous and absorbs everything you put on it. Everything you apply topically to your skin will penetrate and be in your bloodstream within 20 minutes. Because what you put on your skin will end up in your body, treat your skin well and your body will feel and look its best.

Non-toxic products work better. They don't disrupt the natural state of your skin or body, and the bottom-line is that they are safer to use. Other products containing chemicals can cause irritations and sometimes serious medical issues.

When I was younger and didn't know any better I would be taken in by the celebrity endorsements and the beautiful packaging (of course at a great expense) of many skin-care products. I didn't realize the damage I was doing to my skin with these products.

Fortunately for me, I learned about organic products in time to save both my skin and my health. My hope for you is that after reading this book it will be a wake-up call for you to treat your skin better. Let's face it, you can't change just one thing and expect your lifetime of destruction to reverse overnight. You must make a conscious effort and take your health seriously. You have only one body and one life. Now is the time to take control.

Start by making conscious decisions about what you are going to eat, how much exercise you are going to get, and what products you are going to use on your body. To me, going organic is the only way. You can nourish your skin, fight the signs of aging, and stay healthier – all by going organic. Try it. I know you will become a believer, too. Treat yourself to the best skin care because you are worth every penny.

ABOUT SANTIZERS

Some of you may be aware that the Food and Drug Administration is coming down hard on antibacterial products. Because of the importance of this issue I am forwarding to you verbatim an article written by the FDA regarding chemicals in products you purchase over the counter:

When you buy soaps and body washes, do you reach for the bar or bottle labeled 'antibacterial'? Are you thinking that these products, in addition to keeping you clean, will reduce your risk of getting sick or passing on germs to others?

Not necessarily, according to experts at the FDA.

Every day, consumers use antibacterial soaps and body washes at home, work, school, and in other public settings. Especially because so many consumers use them, the FDA believes there should be clearly demonstrated benefits to balance any potential risks.

In fact, there currently is no evidence that over-the-counter (OTC) antibacterial soap products are any more effective at preventing illness than washing with plain soap and water, says Colleen Rogers, Ph.D., a lead microbiologist at FDA

Moreover, antibacterial soap products contain chemical ingredients, such as triclosan and triclocarban, which may carry unnecessary risks given that their benefits are unproven.

"New data suggest that the risks associated with long-term, daily use of antibacterial soaps may outweigh the benefits," Rogers says. "There are indications that certain ingredients in these soaps may contribute to bacterial resistance to antibiotics, and may have unanticipated hormonal effects that are of concern to FDA."

This article was printed on Dec. 19, 2013 on the FDA's website and the news also aired on radio and television.

We at Nourish Skin Care Products want you to be aware that harsh chemicals used on your skin topically could potentially have long-term side effects. The best and most safe way to care for your skin is by using nature's own moisturizers like Nourish Skin Care Products, which are organic and botanical. They will give your skin a natural, healthy, and lustrous glow.

Chapter 4

...

CARING FOR YOUR SKIN

NOT EVERYONE IS BLESSED WITH naturally beautiful skin. Some of the lucky ones are gifted with good genes and it is fairly effortless for them to look beautiful and ageless.

Beauty and beautiful skin unfortunately has been defined by what you see in the movies and on television. Don't always believe what you see, in most cases those models and stars have much help with modern technology and their imperfections are being erased by the computers they use to edit their pictures. Surprisingly, you probably would not recognize most of those celebrities if you saw them on the street because they look completely different without the help of all their touch-ups.

People today also are using a wide variety of skin care products, some with chemicals and some natural or organic brands. Some people seem to get by using anything on their skin and still look marvelous. However, others have severe reactions to those products. Even those who have no reactions are jeopardizing their bodies by allowing chemicals into their bloodstream. For those of you with delicate or problematic skin, you should always be aware of the irritating chemicals hidden in most of the so-called miracle products on the market today.

People have different skin conditions, and unbelievably, some of the conditions are caused by the way they are treating or not treating their skin. For example, people with oily skin (which is more prone to acne) may worsen their condition by over cleansing. They should be washing their skin morning and night time with a mild cleanser. When you cleanse more often, your oiliness or acne could worsen. When you remove the natural acid mantle that protects your skin, your body will try to compensate by producing excess amounts of oil.

When you have extra sensitive skin, it is important to use scent-free or hypoallergenic cleansers. Many scents are alcohol-based and therefore very drying and irritating to the skin. I recommend using an all-natural or organic skin cleanser for this type of skin.

Skin care should be an important part of everyone's body maintenance routine, but skin care products at the department store's cosmetic counter can end up costing a small fortune. More expensive products tend to have more expensive packaging to convey the idea you are buying something special.

Affordable skin care products are not necessarily of low quality; effective ingredients are expensive. The problem with most high-end companies is they spend millions of dollars on advertisement strategies and celebrity endorsements. These costs are built into the cost of their products.

You need to learn the secret of how to find effective, affordable skin care that works. Natural, affordable skin care brands are the safest option.

TIPS TO HELP YOU

* **Protect** – Protect your skin against the damage of free radicals. Read your ingredients to know the benefits provided within the bottle.

* **Chemicals in the formula** – Do not buy products containing harsh chemicals, such as paraben, sulfates, alcohols, fragrances, and glycol. Those ingredients can cause dry skin, allergic reactions, and premature aging. Avoid brands made with synthetic ingredients.

* **Revitalize** – The product you choose should make your skin look smooth, younger, and illuminated. Natural ingredients should be there to make your skin look supple and velvet-like without obstructing the pores.

We at Nourish Your Skin have taken all the above into consideration. It was our goal to bring everyone a quality product that works and also fits into their budget. We do not advertise, but have chosen to sell our products woman to woman and friend to friend.

KEEP YOUR SKIN HAPPY

It is very important to keep your skin clean. Keeping your hands clean is especially important because your hands can spread germs to the skin on other parts of your body.

When washing your hands, use warm water. Wet your hands, then lather up with a mild soap. You should lather and rub everywhere, including the palms, the wrists, between the fingers, and under the nails. Rinse well, dry thoroughly with a clean towel, and you're done.

You'll also want to use water that's warm, not too hot, when you take a shower or bath, water that is too hot can dehydrate your skin. Use a gentle soap to clean your body. Don't forget under your arms and behind your ears! Your face needs attention, especially as you enter puberty and the skin on your face gets oilier. It's a good idea to wash your face once or twice daily with warm water and a mild cleanser. You do not need to scrub hard.

Your body produces its own moisturizer, the oil called sebum that we mentioned previously. It forms a protective layer over your skin. If you wash too much of this off, your skin is likely to feel dry and itchy. If you do have dry, flaky, or itchy skin, you might use a moisturizer. When choosing a moisturizer, look for a moisturizer that is preferably fragrance free.

With pimples, you might think that scrubbing your face is the way to get rid of them. But actually, your skin will be less likely to break out if you clean it gently, using your fingertips, not a rough washcloth. If you have trouble with pimples, talk with your doctor about which cleansers are best.

WHAT ELSE SHOULD YOU DO?
Remember to drink lots of water - your skin loves it.

Regular exercise is good for your skin.

Eat healthy so that your skin gets the vitamins and minerals it needs to carry out all the jobs it must do.

At What Age Should We Start A Skincare Regimen?

Personally, I believe it is never too early to start taking steps to develop a skincare regimen. When children are young is the best time to start good habits that will last their lifetime. Taking care of our skin is as important as flossing and brushing every day and we start teaching those skills to our toddlers.

Below, I have listed the steps to practice for different age groups and how I would recommend taking care of their skin.

Babies / Young Children

As babies, we have the softest skin because it is loaded with healthy collagen and elastin. The skin has plenty of proteins and hyaluronic acid to keep it strong, flexible, and hydrated. We protect our babies by keeping them completely out of the direct sun until they are old enough to begin wearing sunscreen.

By age 4 or 5, as children become capable of handling their own hygiene (toileting, bathing, brushing teeth) they also are ready to learn to wash their faces and moisturize their skin. Start teaching them the importance of using sunscreen to protect their skin from the harmful UV rays that come from being in the sun.

It is important that you teach children the importance of washing away the dirt and grime of each day. Always purchase products that are organic and contain none of the harmful chemicals contained in many over-the-counter cleansers, moisturizers, and sunscreens. Remember that what is applied to the skin also penetrates the skin and goes into your child's bloodstream.

PRETEENS / TEENS

When your child becomes preteen it is even more important to keep the skin clean. Clean skin will help minimize breakouts that come as preteens approach puberty. Oily skin has more of a tendency for breakouts so it is important to wash the skin twice a day to remove dirt, oil, makeup etc. Preteens typically also spend a lot of time in the sun (sports, activities, recess) so don't forget to remind them to use sunscreen daily during these outdoor activities. Preteens also need to get enough sleep, drink enough water, and eat healthy food.

As children hit the teenage years, they need to continue with their basic skincare regimen that you have been teaching them since they were young. Wearing sunscreen, washing their faces, and using moisturizer should now be second nature and part of their daily morning and evening routines. Tell them to beware of too much sunbathing, and keep reminding them to always use sunscreen.

Young Adults

OK, now comes the serious talk about prevention. It is imperative that you take antiaging routines seriously. ALWAYS use sunscreen as a daily routine, and I recommend an SPF 30 or higher. Make sure you are using a daily moisturizer that is loaded with antioxidants and hyaluronic acid. It is time to start using eye crème, keep the skin around your eyes always moist to prevent early wrinkles. If your skin is already showing signs of aging due to soaking in the sun during your younger years, you can add a topical antioxidant like vitamin C serum.

Just to make clear, boys have similar skin conditions as girls and it is just as important that they also follow this same skin regimen. Skin is skin and no matter what your gender, you need to take care of it.

CHILDREN AND SKINCARE

Ingredients in products that are applied topically may penetrate the skin and enter the small blood vessels located just below the surface of the skin, and this can be detrimental for children. The blood then circulates the chemicals through the entire body. Most people use skincare products daily, which magnifies the danger of exposure to harmful ingredients, especially for children.

THINK OF YOUR CHILDREN

Children have a much smaller surface area than adults and therefore harmful chemicals can be more concentrated and potentially more dangerous to them. We love our children above all and we want to protect them from any potential harm. We wish for them happy and healthy lives. So, when it comes to skin protection and caring for the skin, it is important to use the best products available. When choosing healthy products, it is important to read your ingredients, use only safe and healthy ingredients to protect your child from irritants, allergens, or harmful chemicals. Avoid the following:

Fragrances

Many fragrances are made up of chemicals and alcohols, which in many cases irritate asthma, allergies, and bring on migraine headaches. Natural scents may still be an irritant for those with sensitive skin. I recommend for your precious child a fragrance-free product.

Parabens

A definite no-no!! Parabens are used to prevent the growth of bacteria in cosmetic products and can be absorbed through the skin, blood, and digestive system. They have been found in biopsies from breast tumors.

SLS/SLES

These sulfates are found in more than 90 percent of personal care products. They break down your skin's moisture barrier, leading to dry skin.

Formaldehyde

Formaldehyde is a toxic preservative and not something you want in your skin care nor do you want your products releasing this dangerous compound into your skin. Check your labels, whether natural or not.

Read your labels!! Protect your children from these harmful ingredients!!

BELOW ARE LISTED THE DEFINITE YESES TO USE FOR CHILDREN:

* Use a gentle, organic fragrance-free body wash and shampoo
* Use fragrance-free, organic, and chemical-free baby wipes
* Use organic fragrance-free body lotion
* Use cornstarch-based, talc-free powder
* Use broad-spectrum sunscreen rated Sun Protection Factor (SPF) of 25 or greater with micronized zinc oxide as the active ingredient.
* Keep your child's delicate skin out of the sunlight as much as possible. Ask your pediatrician at what age is safe for you to start applying sunscreen. Until the age your doctor recommends, keep your child's delicate skin covered as much as possible.

YOUR CHILD IS GROWING UP

Explain to maturing children the importance of caring for their skin, that it is not just there to keep their insides from falling out. Your children need to know their skin is the largest organ of their bodies and they only get one shot at taking care of it. Their skin is there to protect them from infections and keep them from getting sick. If they take good care of their skin now, they will ward off wrinkles and skin cancers as they get older.

MEN GET WRINKLES, TOO

Men need to take care of their skin as well as women. There are great benefits for those men who have a basic skin-care routine. If your skin is healthy you will look younger longer and therefore more attractive. You will feel better about yourself, giving self-confidence a boost. With a regular skin-care routine you will have fewer breakouts, make shaving easier and experience fewer ingrown hairs.

BAR SOAP VERSUS LIQUID CLEANSER

Studies show that most men prefer bar soap to liquid cleansers. That works. However, there are many choices of organic bar soaps to choose from in the marketplace. Look for a bar soap rich in vitamin E, jojoba oil, or olive oil. Normal bar soaps tend to dry out the skin. If your skin feels tight or itchy after using your normal bar soap, you should consider changing to a milder, more moisturizing liquid cleanser.

MEN AND SKIN CANCER

Studies show that if you are a Caucasian male over the age of 50, you need to know that skin cancer is the No. 1 form of cancer in this age group. However, regardless of what your skin type is, everyone has issues with dry skin, especially in the winter months.

The most common reason for this is that most men spend time outdoors exposing themselves to ultraviolet radiation from the sun without protection.

Antioxidants are what protect the skin from damage as a result of free radicals. Free radicals cause cell damage and many forms of cancer are believed to be due to the reactions between DNA and free radicals leading to malignancy.

HOW SHOULD MEN HELP TO PREVENT SKIN CANCER AND DRY SKIN?

Never use products containing irritants such as alcohol, menthol, peppermint, or too much fragrance (either synthetic or natural). Unfortunately, most men's products contain irritants, so be careful.

Follow a simple routine. Skin has certain needs in order to stay healthy.

1. Cleanse the skin thoroughly with a non-drying soap, we recommend Nourish Body Wash for your body and Nourish Milk Facial Cleanser for your face.

2. Maintain hydration and moisture in the skin. When skin dries out and is over exposed to ultra-violet radiation it is subject to sun damage. To insure a beautiful moisturized skin we recommend Nourish Body Lotion and Nourish Body Oil.

3. Aftershave lotions and toners contain astringents that tighten the skin, narrowing the pores and creating a firmer skin barrier. Witch hazel is an inexpensive solution that can be used to take the puffiness out of lower eyelids. Avoid toners and astringents that contain alcohol, which causes dryness. Enjoy Nourish Your Skin Products Ultra Moisturizing Toner (which contains witch hazel) that not only tightens and tones, but moisturizes as well.

Chapter 5

• • •

How to Slow Down the Aging Process

What we <u>can</u> do to slow down the natural aging process

THE SECRET TO A YOUNGER looking you lies in how you take care of your body and skin. Just a quick synopsis on what you can expect and the kinds of changes your skin will experience in your lifetime and some simple steps in fighting the aging process.

<u>In Your 20s</u> Your skin generally looks healthy. You may develop some freckles that appear in the summer and fade in the winter. The most common problems in this age group are acne, blackheads, and large pores. This is when to start a careful and consistent skin-care routine.

<u>In Your 30s</u> Mild sun damage starts to show in your face and neck areas. You may notice the beginnings of crow's-feet and fine lines, but these generally go away when the face is relaxed. If you haven't already, implement a daily skin-care regimen that protects and moisturizes your skin.

<u>In Your 40s</u> Sun spots and blotchiness on the neck and chest may become more prominent. Crow's-feet

and smile lines now remain visible even when your face is relaxed. Protection and moisturizing are essential now to maintaining healthier skin, and fighting the aging process.

IN YOUR 50S You may notice deeper wrinkles on your forehead and around your mouth as well as the appearance of new wrinkles on your cheeks as well as on your upper lip. Your skin is starting to thin. Sun spots get larger and appear in other places such as your arms, legs, and the backs of your hands. Drinking water, maintaining physical activity, and consistent daily skin care will help minimize the impact of aging.

IN YOUR 60S AND BEYOND With the continued loss of collagen, your skin may begin to sag, especially along the neck and jawline as well as bruise more easily. Dry skin is also a major concern for women in their 60s and 70s. Deep moisturizing, drinking water, maintaining a healthy lifestyle of a nutritious diet and regular exercise will slow this process, regardless of age.

The secret to combatting the above stages in aging are simple and easy to follow.

THERE ARE ONLY THREE SIMPLE STEPS TO HEALTHIER, YOUNGER, AND MORE VIBRANT-LOOKING SKIN.

1. **CLEANSE** – Always use a mild cleanser when bathing. Never use hot water because it will remove natural oils on the surface of your skin and leave you dry and itchy.

2. **MOISTURIZE** – While your skin is still moist apply a moisturizer that is natural and ultra-rich. Check your labels; use products that contain no alcohol.

3. **PROTECT** – Use a natural-based sun-screen. Micronized Zinc Oxide is a great natural base for sun-screen.

Using these three simple steps will help you to have a younger, healthier, and happier skin for a lifetime.

WHY WE GET WRINKLES

AND MORE IMPORTANTLY WHAT CAN WE DO TO LESSEN THEM.

Wrinkles are creases in the skin. Some are fine lines, while others are deep folds. Wrinkles usually appear as we age. Listed below are some of the causes:

1. Facial expressions
2. Genetics
3. Dehydration
4. Sun damage
5. Smoking and excessive use of alcohol
6. Possibly some medications

Wrinkles tend to appear first on body parts that are most exposed to the sun such as the face, neck, back of the hands and arms.

Wrinkles are a natural part of the aging process. As we get older, our skin gets thinner, drier, and less elastic. We need to take more care to delay the results of the list above. When you smile or frown or squint you are using a facial muscle under the skin, which forms a groove. When a person is young the skin tends to spring back, but as we age, and the skin loses some of its elasticity, those grooves tend to be more permanent.

Genetics is something we have no control over. Some of us are lucky and some not so lucky. The lucky ones can thank their ancestors for their generous gift, others oh well…. We must work to have beautiful skin.

THERE ARE SOME OF THE ABOVE WE DO HAVE CONTROL OVER, TO A DEGREE.
Dehydration, for example, we can improve simply by drinking plenty of water. By cutting your alcohol consumption, you also will lessen dehydration of the skin.

Sun damage can be lessened by limited exposure to ultraviolet (UV) light. Limit or end your exposure to the sun by avoiding sunbathing and stopping the use of tanning beds. Both of these options will not only help you from not developing early wrinkles but lessen the chances of skin cancer. UV light can break down the collagen and elastin fibers in your skin. These fibers form the skin's connective tissue under the surface and provide support for skin. When you break down this layer, it causes your skin to become not only weak but less flexible. Your skin will then start to sag and wrinkles will appear.

Eliminating smoking also will help to slow down the aging process. Smoking reduces blood supply to the skin, which accelerates aging.

For fine-line wrinkles, uneven skin tone, or rough skin a topical solution is available. Vitamin C is available in cream or serum formulas. Before using vitamin creams, it is best to consult with your dermatologist or doctor because some people could be allergic to them. In most cases, the adverse effects could be dryness, itching, or a burning sensation.

Be diligent about keeping your skin well fed with a good organic oil, lotion, or both. Always remove your makeup before retiring every night, and drink lots of water.

For more severe issues, you can consult your physician about different cosmetic surgeries or other medical procedures. Some of the options are dermabrasion, laser therapy, chemical peels, fillers, or face lifts.

Remember, aging is a natural process and eventually everybody will get wrinkles. You can lengthen the time you are wrinkle free but not eliminate forever the dreaded wrinkles.

WHAT IS CREPEY SKIN?

Well, the quick and easy answer to that question is simple. The word crepey is used to describe skin that looks like crepe paper, which has a thin, wrinkled texture. When caring for skin, we cannot concentrate solely on our faces because our skin also is aging from the neck down. As skin matures the netting that keeps the skin smooth dries out, which creates the crepey look.

As the body slows down the production of elastin and collagen -- the proteins that allow the skin to stretch and contract -- the skin will begin to sag and wrinkle, typically after age 40. You will notice the most significant changes near the knees, elbows, chest, feet, neck, and hands. Take careful care of your skin, however, and you won't look in a mirror and see aged, crepey skin. There are many healthy ways to avoid it.

HOW CAN WE IMPROVE CREPEY SKIN?

Crepey skin is creepy, so let's do something to change it. Let's turn back the clock and revive your dry, dull skin. As we age, skin feels drier because the body stops producing as many new skin cells and no longer retains the moisture your skin needs. The skin also will slow down the production of the oils that help feed and plump the collagen and elastin in your skin. You can visibly plump and give your skin volume by removing dry skin cells and moisturizing your skin.

Our tips:

First: Never use over-the-counter soap or body wash that contains harsh ingredients such as sulfates.

Second: Use an organic body scrub to wash away dry, dead skin.

Third: Apply an organic skin revitalizer that is rich in hydrators such as coconut oil, olive oil, cocoa butter, shea butter, vitamin E and hyaluronic acid.

Fourth: Always use an organic sunscreen whenever you are exposing your skin to the sun. My recommendation would be to use a sunscreen containing micronized zinc oxide as the main sun-blocking ingredient.

LOVE THE SKIN YOU'RE IN, AND YOU WON'T HAVE TO LOOK OLD. BRING OUT YOUR NATURAL BEAUTY AND WEAR YOUR SKIN WITH CONFIDENCE.

7 SKIN-CARE RESOLUTIONS TO MAKE NOW

Admit it, you still occasionally sleep in your makeup, sometimes forget to use sun screen, or put off seeing your dermatologist for a full body skin check-up. We all slip from our routines on occasion, but if you really want to love your skin, we suggest adopting this seven-step regimen:

1. MOISTURIZE AFTER SHOWERING

We all know a warm shower strips skin of its natural oils. We must moisturize after bathing with an organic moisturizer, but we sometimes forget. One easy fix: Keep the body lotion in the shower. Seeing it will remind you to apply it when your skin is damp, within ten minutes of turning off the water.

2. WEAR SUNSCREEN EVERY DAY

Dermatologists will tell you to wear sunscreen every day with a minimum SPF of 30 and reapply as needed. Always use an organic sunscreen, preferably with micronized zinc oxide as the active ingredient. Some sunscreen lotion comes in wipes or sprays for easier application.

3. REMOVE YOUR MAKEUP EVERY NIGHT

You know that makeup can mix with skin oils and dirt to cause pimples. But at the end of the day you are just too tired to take the time to wash. Avoid this situation by washing your face as soon as you get home with an organic milk cleanser. If that is still too tiring then use an organic cleansing pad to simply wipe it off.

4. EXFOLIATE REGULARLY

A baby's skin replenishes itself completely every 14 days, but by age 30, an adult takes a full 28 days to replenish skin. With all that extra time, skin cells have a chance to dry out and lose luster—unless you jump-start the renewal process by exfoliating. Use a gentle organic face scrub once or twice a week.

5. TREAT YOUR HANDS WITH CARE

To keep both your nails and hands from dehydrating, forgo antibacterial gels and instead choose organic moisturizing lotions. Do not use soaps with sulfates in their formulations. When applying sunscreen don't forget your hands. Keep a good supply in your house and the glovebox of your car. Even with UV-protective auto glass, the damaging rays penetrate and will age your face and hands.

6. CLEAN YOUR MAKEUP BRUSHES

Makeup and skin oils build up in your brushes creating a breeding ground for bacteria that can cause irritation. Make-up brushes should be cleaned once a week, but most of us don't. Wash your brushes monthly with a liquid hand soap or baby shampoo and lukewarm water (hot water can cause bristles to fall out), then rinse well, squeeze out the excess water, reshape, and allow the brushes to dry thoroughly by balancing them over the sink. Weekly, spritz them with an antibacterial and dry with a tissue.

7. DON'T PICK AT YOUR FACE

Yes, it's tempting to squeeze a pimple, but just the act of touching your face with your fingers brings pore-clogging oil and dirt to the skin. Keep your hands busy, especially if certain times of day trigger the urge. When you do give in, applying over-the-counter hydrocortisone cream right away can help calm inflammation and prevent long-lasting marks.

AND DON'T FORGET TO MAKE AN APPOINTMENT WITH YOUR DERMATOLOGIST TO CHECK FOR ANY CHANGES IN YOUR SKIN OR MOLES YOU MAY HAVE.

Chapter 6

• • •

The Importance of Good Nutrition and Exercise; You Are What You Eat!

As we have mentioned before, your skin is the largest organ of your body and you need to take care of it. The old cliché says, "beauty is only skin deep," but that's not true either literally or figuratively. Skin beauty does come from the inside because there is a definite connection between nutrition and skin condition.

As babies, we are born with plenty of collagen, which is why as youngsters we have firm, resilient skin. As we mature, our collagen production slows down so our skin gets thinner and less elastic, which makes us more prone to wrinkling. A proper diet will help fight this process and keep our skin looking younger and smoother for a longer period.

How Important is Breakfast?

Breakfast is a critical meal because it gets you going after an overnight fast. It influences our whole being during the day.

Rush-hour mornings can be a time crunch time for many of us. However, no matter how busy you are it is important to take a few extra minutes to fuel your body so you have energy for the rest of the day. Some nutritionists recommend eating breakfast about one hour after waking because our bodies are craving energy right away and waiting too long may make us overeat, therefore causing weight gain.

What you eat is important. I am not recommending a cup of coffee and a doughnut or some of the well-known sugary cereals. Eat a balanced meal for breakfast, as you would for any other meal.

Like some of you, sometimes I am just too lazy or too hurried to cook breakfast. I have discovered a quick and easy breakfast dish that is nutritious and delicious. You might like it, also. You make it the night before and refrigerate it overnight and your breakfast is ready in the morning.

OVERNIGHT OATMEAL

½ cup organic old-fashioned oatmeal (do not cook)

½ cup milk (your choice of milk, but unsweetened almond milk or unsweetened coconut milk is recommended)

1 teaspoon organic sugar, you also may use an equivalent Stevia serving or 1/16 to ½ teaspoon of (sugar substitute) xylitol (to your taste)

1 teaspoon pure vanilla

½ cup your choice of fresh fruit (fruit may be eliminated if you are watching your sugar intake).

1 teaspoon chia seeds

Mix oats, milk, sugar, and vanilla together is 8-oz. Mason jar

Place fruit on top and sprinkle with chia seeds. Refrigerate overnight.

Another choice for a healthy breakfast provided by Lisa Henss that eliminates the sugar follows:

Lisa's Egg Muffins

12 eggs

1-2 cups grated, low-fat cheese (use less cheese if using meat)

3 small, green cnions, diced

Optional chopped veggies such as blanched broccoli, red pepper, zucchini, mushrooms, crumbled cooked turkey sausage.

Preheat oven to 375 F. Use regular or silicone muffin pan, 12-muffin size. Put two paper liners into each slot. In the bottom of the muffin cups, layer your choice of any the following but limit to the muffin cup being 2/3 full:

- diced meat
- vegetables
- cheese
- or green onions.

Break eggs into a large measuring bowl with pour spout, and beat well. Pour eggs into each muffin cup until each is 3/4 full. You may stir slightly with a fork to dampen the other ingredients. Bake 25 to 35 minutes, or until muffins have risen and are slightly browned and set.

Muffins will keep more than a week in the refrigerator. Egg muffins can be frozen and re-heated but they taste their best when fresh or just refrigerated.

A well-balanced diet is important in maintaining healthy skin as well as a healthy body. It is important to get plenty of protein and good fats. Protein is the natural way to build collagen in your body. Collagen helps to keep your skin firm and toned.

EXAMPLES OF PROTEINS:

Turkey or chicken breast	Both birds consist mostly of protein, with very little fat and calories. They also taste delicious.
Meats	Lean beef is very high in protein, and tastes also is loaded with highly bio-available iron, vitamin B12 and numerous other nutrients.
Eggs	Eggs are a complete source of protein, and contain biotin, an essential vitamin that protects against dry skin.
Cottage Cheese	It is loaded with calcium, phosphorus, selenium, vitamin B12, riboflavin (vitamin B2) and various other nutrients.
Oats	Oats are among the healthiest grains on the planet. They are loaded with healthy fibers, magnesium, manganese, thiamin (vitamin B1) and several other nutrients.
Fish	Salmon contains astaxanthin, a keto-carotenoid that improves skin elasticity, so you'll have fewer fine lines.

Beans	They are high in <u>fiber</u>, magnesium, potassium, iron, folate, copper, manganese and various other nutrients.
Almonds	They are loaded with important nutrients, including fiber, vitamin E, manganese and magnesium.
Pumpkin Seeds	They are incredibly high in many nutrients, including iron, magnesium and zinc.

LET'S TALK ABOUT CARBOHYDRATES

Carbohydrates, commonly known as carbs, are an essential part of a healthy diet because they are the body's primary source of energy. However, there are different types of carbohydrates. Some are better for you than others. If you have a sweet tooth (like I do), you tend to think of cakes, cookies, candies, etc. Let me explain the difference between good carbs and bad carbs. How do you know which is which? Carbs can be either simple (bad) or complex (good).

EXAMPLES OF SIMPLE (BAD) CARBS:

Added sugar is the single worst ingredient in the modern diet, and it finds its way into all types of foods we eat. Be aware of hidden sugar by reading nutrition labels carefully.

Simple carbs are easy to digest, added sugars (like sucrose and high fructose corn syrup) contain a whole bunch of calories with but no essential nutrients. When reading the nutrition label, avoid foods high in sugar and low in fiber. Fruits and some vegetables also fall into the simple carb arena, so eating too much can also affect sugar levels and weight gain. However, the fiber in fruits and vegetables also offsets the way that the body processes their sugars and slows down digestion, making them more like complex carbohydrates and less likely to cause wild fluctuations in blood-sugar levels. They are healthier than processed sugar, but you should still be aware of how many fruits you eat, and starchy vegetables such as corn or potatoes.

The following are simple carbs that if not eliminated from your diet should be eaten in limited quantities or only as a treat:

* Soft drinks
* Fruit drinks
* Candies
* Jams and jellies
* Pastries and desserts

- Syrups
- Sugar (yes, brown sugar, also)

The simple carbs below are better choices, but still should be eaten sparingly:

- White rice, white bread, and white pasta
- Potatoes (which are technically a complex carb, but act more like simple carbs in the body)
- Fruits
- Some vegetables such as corn

EXAMPLES OF COMPLEX (GOOD) CARBOHYDRATES:

Complex carbs are made of sugar molecules strung together. They are often rich in fiber. Complex carbs are generally found in whole plant foods, making them higher in vitamins and minerals.

Consuming complex carbs is important to ensure the body has what it needs to perform at its optimum level. Complex carbs take a longer time to digest and are the key to fulfilling hunger as well as providing a long-lasting source of energy.

The following complex carbs are examples of healthy choices to give you a strong healthy body, and healthy skin:

* Green vegetables
* Whole grains and foods made from them such as oatmeal, pasta and sprouted whole-grain breads.
* Sweet potatoes and squash
* Beans, lentils, and peas
* Full fat dairy (low fat has added sugar)
* Nuts and seeds
* Granny Smith apples, and all berries

Try making some substitutions from simple carbs to complex carbs, such as:

* Instead of white bread and pasta try sprouted whole grain bread and whole grain pasta.
* Instead of eating chips try eating raw vegetables
* Instead of white rice try eating more beans (especially black beans).

HEALTHY FOODS TO EAT:

Protein	Vegetables	Complex Carbs
Buffalo meat	Artichoke	Granny Smith
Chicken breast	Asparagus	Apples
Crab	Broccoli	Barley
Eggs	Brussel	Beans
Haddock	sprouts	Corn
Lean ground	Cabbage	Couscous
beef	Carrots	Full fat yogurt
& turkey	Cauliflower	Full fat milk
Lean Ham	Celery	High fiber cereal
Lobster	Cucumber	Kashi
Full fat cottage	Green beans	Lentils
cheese	Green	Melon
Orange Roughy	peppers	Oatmeal
Salmon	Lettuce	Orange
Shrimp	Zucchini	Potato
Swordfish	Mushrooms	Pumpkin
Sprouted Grains	Onion	Steamed brown
Trout	Peas	rice
Tuna	Spinach	Sweet potato
Turkey bacon		All Berries
Quinoa		Squash

Good fats

Contrary to what we have been told in the past, good fats are essential to your good health and a healthy skin. Good fats have a high nutritional value and are extremely good for you.

Daily doses of good fat are important for your organs to function properly. Without enough fat in your diet your energy levels may drag and your ability to focus may be diminished because you always feel hungry. Always being hungry leads to irritability and depression.

It is important to understand which fats are considered healthy and what nutrients in fatty foods can help to keep you healthy. The following are some examples of healthy, fatty foods:

Avocados are extremely high in fat, but they contain a monounsaturated fat that is great for your body. Avocados are high in calories, but they're also high in fiber and potassium. They've been shown to lower bad and raise good blood cholesterol, two important factors in cardiovascular health. This fruit (yes, it's a fruit) also contains antioxidants, one of which promotes good eye health.

OLIVE OIL is very healthy and is rich in nutrients. Olive oil is also rich in monounsaturated fat. Some of the benefits of olive oil are reducing the risk of some cancers, lowering blood pressure, and helping to lower the risk of heart disease.

SALMON is another fatty food that has mega health benefits and is packed full of nutrients. Salmon is high in protein and omega-3 fatty acids. Salmon is a key food to help reduce the risk of heart disease. Salmon contributes to brain and joint health, and it also lowers the risk of some types of cancers, depression, and Alzheimer's disease.

EGGS contain many vitamins, HDL (good cholesterol), and antioxidants, they are also a healthy source of protein. The nutrients in eggs may protect and maintain eye health, lower the risk of heart disease and stroke.

NUTS offer many health benefits. Nuts are full of monounsaturated fats and omega-3 fatty acids. According to the Mayo Clinic, monounsaturated fatty acids can help reduce the risk of heart disease by improving heart-related risks like lowering cholesterol and possibly normalizing blood clotting.

COCONUTS are a fatty food. Coconuts have many health benefits and can be used in a variety of ways. You may use coconut as an oil, raw coconut, or coconut flakes, in all forms they are beneficial to your health. Coconut oil is higher in HDL cholesterol (the good kind). Replace your butter or other oils with the benefits of the healthy coconut or just eat it as a snack.

FLAXSEED is food that is rich in omega-3 fatty acids, fiber, and phytochemicals. The high amount of nutrients within flaxseeds have been proven to help improve health in several different ways. You can add a small amount to your shakes or smoothies. Health benefits include reduced blood pressure, lowered bad cholesterol, and better digestion.

PEANUT BUTTER is a fatty food that offers many health benefits because it's high in potassium, protein, fiber, and unsaturated fats (the good fat). It can decrease the risk of heart disease and diabetes, reduce abdominal fat, and keep you full for longer. Use in the raw form to get the maximum benefit.

ALMOND BUTTER is a food that is high in healthy fats. Almond butter helps to improve bone health and energy. It reduces the risk of heart disease and protects your skin. When purchasing always look for the organic version that has no sugar nor sodium.

DARK CHOCOLATE Yum! Dark chocolate is rich in antioxidants and fiber, which helps reduce the risk of heart disease, protects skin, and lowers bad cholesterol. To be considered dark chocolate it must be at least 70 percent cocoa.

Vitamins That Keep Your Skin Healthy

Is your skin dry, your lips chapped, and your hair lacking luster? It could be that you are low in nutrients such as vitamins, minerals, and anti-oxidants. I have listed below some of the more important vitamins that will help your body and skin thrive. However, with any vitamins, minerals, or anti-oxidants, I always recommend talking with your doctor or nutritionist to make sure that they don't interfere with any medications you are taking. You have the power to give yourself younger-looking skin and a healthier body just by using some of the tricks in this book.

Biotin

Has been found to effectively treat brittle nails. If you have soft, dry, weak, and easily breakable nails that show lines or striations in the nail plate or have fingernail splitting, try adding biotin to your diet.

Some food sources for biotin include: nuts, sunflower seeds, legumes, cauliflower, bananas, and avocados.

Vitamin A (Beta-Carotene)

Vitamin A is an essential part in the development of an effective physical and water barrier function in the skin. Some food sources for Vitamin A include: sweet potatoes, carrots, spinach, romaine lettuce, butternut squash, cantaloupe, red peppers, dried apricots, peas, and broccoli.

Vitamin C

Centuries ago sailors discovered the key to avoiding scurvy, eating citrus high in Vitamin C while on long voyages. Vitamin C also has a vital role in maintaining the health of your skin. It can improve hair growth, fight dandruff, and stop hair loss. Your skin will appear to have less dryness and appear tighter after a short period of time. Vitamin C is key to the production of collagen that gives the skin its firmness and strength. It also helps your skin repair itself.

Some Vitamin C food sources would be oranges, strawberries and limes.

Vitamin E

Like Vitamin C, Vitamin E is a powerful antioxidant that helps fight free-radical damage that leads to fine lines. Because Vitamin E is fat-soluble it is best to take it in the gel cap form. Again, always check with your primary care doctor to see if this vitamin is right for you.

Some Vitamin E food sources would be avocado, olive oil and wheat germ.

OMEGA-3 FATTY ACIDS

Omega-3's regulate oil production and help keep your skin moisturized. Another benefit is that they delay the skin's aging process. Omega-3's can make your hair shine, keep your hair moisturized and your scalp from flaking. Some Omega-3 food sources are salmon, sardines, and mackerel.

VITAMIN B

B vitamins are essential for nurturing cells throughout the body, including skin cells. Biotin is a B vitamin that supports your skin, nerves, lessons hair loss and encourages nail growth. Vitamin B deficiency can lead to dry, itchy skin.

Some vitamin B and biotin food sources are chicken, eggs, fortified grain products, peanut butter, walnuts, and bananas.

Vitamin D3

This is another of the best vitamins for hair, skin, and nails. It acts to regulate the production of keratin, the main component in hair, skin, and nails. These effects have led to the use of vitamin D for the treatment of psoriasis. Some vitamin D3 food sources include: Fish, milk, and mushrooms.

Zinc

Concentrations are high in the skin and deficiency of this mineral leads to dermatitis and other skin disorders.

Some Zinc food sources include: Oysters, lobster, crab, beef, pork, chicken, lentils, nuts, seeds, milk, dairy foods, and dark chocolate.

Keep Your Body Strong With Exercise

Why exercise is important

To maintain a healthy lifestyle, it is very important to exercise. Exercise may prevent many various health issues as well as giving you strength and energy. Exercise will help you retain a healthy body weight and reduce your stress levels.

There are many benefits in adding exercise to your regular routine. You may reduce your risk for heart disease, reduce your high blood pressure, diabetes, and obesity.

As we age we have a higher risk of falls, with exercise you keep yourself flexible and you move around with more ease. I find that I also have much improvement in my sleep patterns.

How exercise benefits the skin

If you are exercising correctly you are working up a sweat. When you sweat, your heart works more, your circulation improves and you are speeding up your metabolism. As your circulation increases the built up toxins and impurities are able to exit your body by way of your open skin pores. After you exercise follow up with bathing, and moisturizing to achieve a more nourished skin.

Is exercise for everyone?

Exercise can help you feel better from the inside out

Everyone can benefit from an exercise program. You can begin your program with as little as 12 minutes per day two to three times per week. Exercise at your own pace. If you have a health problem that is being monitored, consult with your doctor before you begin any exercise program. You can slowly work your way to a larger goal of five times per week for up to 30 minutes per day.

If you are having trouble sticking with your program, find a friend to work out with you. When you have a partner, you can motivate each other when one of you isn't in the mood to exercise. It is a great incentive to have someone to share your workouts and celebrate your successes.

There is no excuse not to exercise

The word exercise shouldn't be a scary word. You can exercise from anywhere; it doesn't have to be a fancy gym membership. **It can be free.** Below are some ideas you can use, even if you are traveling. They can be used for any age group by simply modifying the time and repetitions that you do.

The most important thing to remember about exercise is to get your heart rate up. A good way to do that is the 20-second interval method. So, exercise as hard as you are able for 20 seconds then rest for 20 seconds. Continue to do that until your 12 minutes are up. If you follow that rule for the following exercises, you will have a good workout.

Arm Raises/Circles

These exercises can be done from anywhere. You may sit or stand and simply raise your arm horizontal to the floor then lower and raise your arm for as many reps as you set for your goal. You may also add a small hand weight for a more intense workout.

For an additional arm exercise you can do arm circles. Hold your arms out to the side at shoulder height. Rotate your shoulders forward then backward and rotate your arms in various sized circles.

Dancing

Dancing is great exercise. Can be done anywhere, any time of day or night. Fast or slow. Great calorie burner.

Leg Raises

Leg raises can be done either sitting or standing. You can do at work sitting at your desk, watching TV or simply lying in bed.

Leg raises can be done by lifting your leg in front of you to stretch the calf and hamstring muscles, behind you to stretch your quads and glutes or out to the side to work your inner and outer thighs.

Sitting Down and Standing up

Squatting to a sitting position and standing back up again works many muscle groups and is good for your balance. Stand up and sit down a few times. You also can hold a squatting position just above the couch or chair you are about to sit down on.

Stretching

Stretching is something you can do anywhere. Stretching first thing in the morning helps muscle and joint stiffness. Stretching before bed helps you relax your body to promote better sleep. If you stretch a few minutes throughout the day it will help keep your muscles from cramping.

Walking

Walking is very beneficial to the body. You can walk at any pace and receive physical and mental benefits. You may adjust to your own level simply by how much distance, how brisk you walk and the time you spend on your walk.

Chapter 7

• • •

TANNING YEAH OR NAY?

BOTTOM LINE, THERE IS NO SAFE WAY TO GET A TAN

ACCORDING TO THE MELANOMA RESEARCH Foundation (MRF) as many as 90 percent of melanomas are estimated to be caused by ultraviolet (UV) exposure from the sun and from artificial sources such as tanning beds. The World Health Organization's International Agency for Research on Cancer (IARC) classifies tanning beds and tanning lamps in its highest cancer risk category.

DON'T BELIEVE EVERYTHING YOU HEAR

The tanning industry has tried to tell consumers that vitamin D is necessary and that it should be sought from tanning beds. However, the majority of tanning bulbs actually emit UVA radiation, and UVB radiation is needed for the body to produce vitamin D. The fact is, all necessary vitamin D can be found in a healthy diet or from a vitamin supplement. If you are concerned about your vitamin D levels, consult your doctor, not a tanning salon!

THIS IS MIND BLOWING

Research indicates that just one blistering sunburn can double your chances of developing melanoma later in life. In addition, using tanning beds before age 30 increases your risk of developing melanoma by 75 percent. Occasional use of tanning beds triples your chances. Research also suggests the more sessions, hours and years spent tanning, the higher the risk of developing melanoma and other types of skin cancer.

What actually is tanned skin?

Tanned skin is a result of damage to skin cells. Research suggests that the cumulative damage to skin cells can lead to wrinkles, age spots, premature aging and skin cancer.

Intentional UV tanning of any kind, in the sun or in a tanning bed, is never recommended.

How about sunless tanning products?

To reduce the dangers of indoor tanning some manufacturers have manufactured topical sunless tanning products so you can get a tanned appearance without UV exposure. A concern has been noted that dihydroxyacetone (DHA), a commonly used ingredient in sunless tanning products and has been approved by FDA for use in cosmetics and drugs for external application only.

The concern lies in using the product in spray tanning booths, inhalation is usually unavoidable.

Over-the-counter sunless tanning creams and lotions are options for those of you who want to have the appearance of tanned skin while avoiding the risks of UV rays or inhaled DHA.

Why is it necessary to change the color of your skin?

HOW ABOUT, "LOVING THE SKIN YOU'RE IN?"

What is SPF?

Sun Protection Factor (SPF) is simply a number on a scale for rating the degree of protection provided by sunscreens.

SPF numbers have a wide range. These numbers refer to the product's ability to screen out the sun's burning rays. It is difficult to predict the exact number for everyone because it depends on your skin's sensitivity to the sun and how long it takes your skin to burn without applying any sunscreen.

In general, if you are in the sun it takes about 10 minutes to 20 minutes without sunscreen for a person's skin to start burning. An SPF 15 product would prevent skin from burning for 15 times longer – so about 150 to 300 minutes, or about two and half to five hours. However, that doesn't mean you're fully protected for that five hours. Dermatologists highly recommend reapplying sunscreen every two to four hours, as sunscreen can rub off or get washed off in the water if you're at the beach or a pool.

A sunscreen with an SPF 15 blocks about 94 percent of the sun's dangerous rays. SPF 30 products block about 97 percent of such rays, and SPF 45 sunscreen shields against about 98 percent of rays. There's really no need to go any higher.

When it comes to choosing a sunscreen, consider any allergies you may have. "Sunscreens use a variety of chemicals that work to absorb harmful UV rays before they penetrate your skin," according to cancer expert Lisa Fayed. Lisa has a Bachelor of Science degree in Biology with a concentration in biochemistry and molecular biology. She is currently pursuing her MD and plans to practice in gynecologic oncology.

"Some people are sensitive or allergic to certain ingredients, like PABA, and choose to use sunblock instead of sunscreen. In fact, many brands today are a blend of sunscreen and sunblock, so it's important to check the label if you have a sensitivity to certain chemicals."

The chemicals are invisible, but the damage they can cause to your skin and health is anything but subtle. Ultraviolet, or UV, radiation comes from the sun and is just one of the forms of energy that reach earth's surface. UV radiation is a combination of UVA, UVB and UVC rays. UVA rays are the number one cause of long-term skin damage, including wrinkles and skin cancer.

UVB rays can damage skin cells at a molecular level and are the main cause of sunburns, according to the American Cancer Society. They also cause most forms of skin cancer. UVC rays do not pass through earth's atmosphere.

UV rays are strongest during the spring and summer and are most intense between 10 a.m. and 4 p.m. And, just because there's cloud cover, doesn't mean you can't get burned. Some 80 percent of the sun's UV radiation can pass through clouds.

SAFE SUNSCREENS

I recommend using a safe sunscreen with the SPF ingredient to be micronized zinc oxide. There are chemical sunscreens and physical sunscreens, the difference between the two are as follows:

CHEMICAL SUNSCREENS penetrate the skin and can interfere with your hormones and could raise your risk for cancer.

PHYSICAL SUNSCREENS that contain micronized zinc oxide do not pose any danger because they aren't absorbed into your skin.

Physical sunscreens work by providing a physical barrier and blocking out the harmful rays. Micronized zinc oxide will block both UVB and UVA rays. Micronized zinc oxide is an invisible form of zinc that does not leave your skin with a white film and at the same time does not penetrate into your bloodstream. Because it does not absorb into your skin, it will protect your skin for a longer period unless it is wiped off, where chemical sunscreens need to be applied every hour to two hours.

Nourish Your Skin sells a micronized zinc oxide formula with a SPF of 30. Visit www.nourishskincareproducts.com to place an order.

How to Reverse Sun Damage

We all enjoy basking in the sunshine with the summer breeze blowing softly over our skin and soaking up some vitamin C and D, but have you considered the implications of what that is doing to your skin? Well, let me share with you some of the not so nice benefits of too much sun exposure.

Reality is premature aging, wrinkles, brown spots, leathery skin and skin cancer, 90 percent of which are caused by too much sun. Not so pretty, huh? Because sun damage accumulates over time, it is never too late to start a sun protection regime to help or even reverse sun damage to the skin.

First things first. Visit your dermatologist for a complete body check to make sure your skin is free from any skin cancers.

Second, you should protect your skin from the sun before your complexion gets worse. Wear a minimum 30 SPF physical sunscreen with a micronized zinc oxide base when you go out, cover up with clothing that will protect, and try to stay out of the sun at the peak hours of 10-4.

Although most people realize the importance of applying sunscreen when the sun is at its peak, it is not enough to just protect your skin from the sun only in the summer months. Sun protection must be practiced year-round so you can prevent further sun damage and maybe even reverse some of the sun damage caused from past years.

Of course, not all skin damage is reversible or curable but you can try to heal skin that has a bad sunburn or mild skin damage.

Some of the following suggestions may help to protect or reverse some of the negative effects of the sun:

REDUCE EXPOSURE TO THE SUN. Use sunscreen daily with the SPF being 15 or higher. Using sunscreen daily may help to lower your long-term risk of skin cancer. When you reduce your daily sun exposure using sunscreen it gives your skin a break and your immune system time to repair some of the existing damage.

USE TOPICAL VITAMIN C REGULARLY, but remember that overuse of vitamin C can be drying to your skin. Apply organic lotions to counteract this side effect. Why do we recommend organic products? Because many of the over-the-counter products are full of chemicals that can be harmful to your skin as well as your health. Regular use of vitamin C can help to reduce aging or brown spots caused by too much UV exposure.

EXFOLIATE TO REMOVE DEAD SKIN CELLS. Buildup of dead skin cells can make your skin appear blotchy and uneven in color. Removing dead cells will make your skin look healthier, even out the tone, and help the skin to look smoother.

DRINK LOTS OF WATER and use a good organic body oil and lotion to moisturize your skin. Hydrated skin gives the appearance of a much younger, less wrinkled person.

Chapter 8

• • •

SKINCARE PRODUCT INGREDIENTS

CHECK YOUR LABELS

IN GENERAL, MOST PEOPLE ARE not aware of the toxic ingredients present in over-the-counter, personal care products. Many of the beauty supplies and products on store shelves today contain toxic ingredients.

WHY IS THAT?

Easy answer: Because they are cheap and readily available. Are they in the products you currently use? Let's see. Go grab your containers of skin care products and compare them against the following ingredients:

TOXIC INGREDIENTS – THE BAD GUYS

PARABENS -- Parabens are widely used as preservatives that prevent the growth of bacteria, mold, and yeast in cosmetic products. Parabens also possess estrogen-mimicking properties that are associated with an increased risk of breast cancer. These chemicals absorb through the skin and have been identified in biopsy samples from breast tumors.

ALCOHOL, ISOPROPYL (SD-40) -- A very drying irritating solvent and dehydrator that will strip your skin of moisture and destroy your natural immune barrier, making your skin more vulnerable to bacteria. It may promote brown spots and cause premature aging of the skin.

SODIUM LAURYL SULFATE (SLS) and sodium laureth sulfate (SLES) – Both are detergents that pose serious health threats. These chemicals are used in car washes, in garage-floor cleaners, and engine degreasers and -- believe it or not -- 90 percent of personal care products that foam, such as hair mousse or shaving cream.

SYNTHETIC FRAGRANCES -- Synthetic ingredients can contain the presence of up to 4,000 separate ingredients, many toxic or carcinogenic. You could be putting on a concoction that contains tons of chemicals that are hazardous to your health. Fragrances can be found in most products such as perfume, cologne, conditioner, shampoo, body wash, and moisturizers. A safe alternative to fragrance would be organic essential oils.

MINERAL OIL -- This is a petroleum by-product that coats the skin like plastic, clogging the pores. It interferes with the skin's ability to eliminate toxins, promoting acne and other disorders. It slows down skin function and cell development, resulting in premature aging.

TRICLOSAN – This is a popular ingredient in just about any product claiming antibacterial properties. It works well at killing bacteria, which creates the issue that not all bacteria are bad for you. Some experts believe the widespread use of this chemical could give rise to superbugs resistant to antibiotics.

ACRYLAMIDE ALSO KNOWN AS POLYACRYLAMIDE – This is used in facial moisturizers, anti-aging products, color cosmetics, lotions, hair products, sunscreens, and more. It can be absorbed by inhaling it or passing through your skin. This should be treated as a dangerous carcinogen and handled with extreme caution. If it encounters your eyes, it can cause irritation, watering, and inflammation.

PROPYLENE GLYCOL – This is a common cosmetic moisturizer and carrier for fragrance oils. This ingredient may cause dermatitis and skin irritation, and it also may inhibit skin cell growth.

PHENOL CARBOLIC ACID – This is a chemical found in many lotions and skin creams. It can cause circulatory collapse, paralysis, convulsions, coma, and – in extreme cases - death from respiratory failure.

DIOXANE – This an ingredient found in compounds known as PEG, polysorbats, laureth, ethoxylatd alcohols. Dioxane is common in a wide range of personal care products. Dioxane's carcinogenicity was first reported in 1965 and later confirmed in studies including one from the National Cancer Institute in 1978. Nasal passages and liver are the most vulnerable.

TOLUENE - Amazingly, toluene is contained in almost all synthetic perfumes and other fragrances, in nail polishes, cosmetics, and other skin care products. It breaks down the skin's natural protective layer, resulting in rashes and red, dry, itchy skin.

The above ingredients are only a few that are harmful to your health and the environment. Our skin is great at absorbing, which means products that we put on our skin also end up in our bloodstream. When we wash those products off, they go down the drain and enter the water supply, polluting waterways, and harming wildlife.

The good news is you can educate yourself and avoid these dangerous toxins. When shopping, read your labels. There are many fine alternatives to those products on the market that use toxic ingredients. Many are much less expensive, especially when you consider the downside years later when you are suffering from ill health because of their toxicity.

ORGANIC INGREDIENTS – THE GOOD GUYS

When checking your labels remember to look for the good ingredients as well as being aware of the bad. The following is a partial list of "the good guys" and the benefits they represent:

ALOE VERA GEL – A natural moisturizer from the leaves of aloe barbadensis lily plants. This gel has been traditionally used for healing and soothing skin burns, cuts and bruises.

AVOCADO OIL – The sterolins found in avocado oil can reduce blemishes in skin caused by sun damage. Avocado oil, for skin care purposes, helps to increase collagen production naturally. Just a few of the vitamins found in avocado oil for skin rejuvenation include vitamins A, various B vitamins including B1 and B2, vitamin D and E, as well as beta carotene, potassium, and lecithin.

Diseases like eczema and psoriasis, which are known for the dry and itchy conditions they cause, can benefit slightly from avocado oil. For hair, avocado oil comprises of many beneficial nutrients such as protein, copper, magnesium, iron, folic acid, and amino acids. All of these nutrients are vital for hair nourishment and growth. The nutrients in avocado oil benefit the health and growth of all types of hair, particularly dry hair, and other hair types such as afro-textured hair. Mixing avocado oil with other beneficial hair oils, such as olive oil, ensures better hair care.

CHAMOMILE EXTRACT – Chamomile is known for its soothing, healing, and protective properties. The yellow color of chamomile infusion imparts brightness and shine and lightens the color of hair. Rinsing with chamomile also may help reduce or prevent hair loss.

COCONUT OIL - Coconut oil is a natural substance said to offer a host of health benefits. One of the few plant sources of saturated fat, coconut oil contains lauric acid (said to possess antibacterial, antiviral, and antioxidant properties).

GRAPESEED OIL - A natural preservative, grapeseed oil prolongs shelf life, and helps to tighten and tone aging skin. It also contains powerful antioxidants such as vitamins E, C, and A. It is non-comedogenic and anti-inflammatory due to its high linoleic acid properties, and it assists in stabilizing collagen and maintaining elasticity. This may help reduce the appearance of wrinkles, age spots, stretch marks and saggy skin. Moisturizing properties lend a shimmering appearance to the skin. It is a natural preservative. Grapeseed extract contains extremely high levels of free radical fighting antioxidants

HYALURONIC ACID - This natural product helps your skin hold on to its own moisture and remain supple for the longest period possible. It also promotes collagen and elastin in the skin. It can have the effect of temporarily plumping wrinkles and fine lines. Absorbs up to 1,000 times its weight in water.

JAPANESE GREEN TEA - This extract is rich in phenolic antioxidants, which provide antiaging properties. The antioxidant present in green tea helps to clear damage caused to the skin and repairs wrinkles, blemishes, or any other impurities on the skin. Japanese green tea extract also soothes the skin and prevents irritation. According to the U.S. National Library of Medicine, a 2007 study by Korean scientists at the Seoul National University College of Medicine found that epigallocatechin-3-gallat, or EGCG, present in green tea promoted growth of hair follicles and stimulated the human dermal papilla cells to boost hair production.

JOJOBA OIL - This is natural botanical liquid wax obtained from the beans of the jojoba plant, a small shrub that grows in the hot, dry climates of California and Arizona. Native Americans have quietly used jojoba oil for hundreds of years to treat various skin maladies. It protects all the other oils used with it and it protects from rancidity.

Jojoba oil works as a natural moisturizer for your skin and lips. A natural emollient, jojoba oil's similarity to sebum allows it to absorb easily and readily into your skin, making it a gentle skin-softening moisturizer for all skin types. Using it can lead to an improvement in both dandruff and acne. Jojoba oil may improve and relieve an assortment of skin conditions, including psoriasis, chapped skin, sunburn, and eczema. It gives strength to hair and makes strands breakage resistant by providing them with required moisturizer and making them free of split-ends and tangles. New cell growth is promoted that makes the hair stronger and gets rid of dryness and frizz.

SESAME SEED OIL - Contains vitamin E in abundance along with vitamin B complex and vitamin A, which helps nourish and rejuvenate skin. Other beneficial nutrients include phosphorus, copper, calcium, zinc, and magnesium. It is also known to contain potent antioxidants that can be beneficial for reversing skin aging.

SHEA BUTTER - This butter is derived from a tree nut. Its botanical source and long heritage of use in skin therapy renders it valuable in our products. It is soften-ing, soothing, and healing to the skin, and protects skin from the sun's damaging rays. It soothes the skin from sunburn, minor burns, itch due to dry skin, rash, skin cracks, and chafing on feet and hands.

SUNFLOWER SEED OIL - Sunflower seed oil provides protection for the skin as it can be easily absorbed. It offers a protective coating that can help prevent infec-tion and inflammation. Sunflower seed oil is also effec-tive in treating acne. Skin care products, such as body wash, cleansers, and moisturizers often contain sun-flower seed oil because of its natural power to retain skin moisture.

SWEET ALMOND OIL - Almond oil is an excellent emol-lient and moisturizer. As an emollient, it nourishes and softens the skin helping to keep it smooth to the touch. Almond oil is similar in composition to the oil babies excrete to keep their skin and hair healthy.

Above are some of the finest in organic ingredients. Nourish Your Skin Products is proud to report that all the above ingredients can be found in our products.

I always recommend going organic. Safe natu-ral ingredients are becoming more popular in the marketplace as people are getting more educated to the lasting effects of harmful chemicals. If you are ready to embrace the benefits of natural skincare so you can have healthier, younger looking skin without subjecting your face and body to harsh chemicals that may end up doing more harm than good check us out on our website www.nourishskincareproducts.com.

Chapter 9

• • •

TESTIMONIALS

DR. BRYAN HENSS ~ FORT WORTH, TX

I RECOMMEND NOURISH YOUR SKIN products to all of my patients because of their clean non-toxic formulation. In an ever increasingly toxic environment, which leads to increasing rates of chronic, degenerative diseases, it is imperative that every family in my office choose as many non-toxic personal care products as possible. My family and I have been using Nourish for several years and we recommend it to everyone we know! –

KAREN ~ PEORIA, AZ

I'm so glad I was able to make it over to Trilogy for the market event last weekend. I love everything I bought. You were right about the unscented body oil being the right way to go. I use it right out of the shower while my legs are still damp, then put the (unscented) body lotion over it to seal it. Works great. Also, the foot smoother is the best thing ever for my heels; so far, I only used it that afternoon. Since then I've used the oil / lotion combination and heels are still in great condition -- and I've been wearing sandals most of this week! The two products go on so smoothly together and there's no greasiness. A friend and I had pedicures later that day and the guy said my feet were in great condition. HA!

Also, I dearly love the lip balm!! It's the first one I've ever tried that doesn't contribute to the dry lips. It actually heals them if the lipstick dries them out. Will have to get some more of that, too (the green one).

I'll be happy to provide a testimonial for your book and thank you for your efforts to offer pure products.

KIM ~ CENTRALIA, WA

I love the Nourish products!!! I have horrible skin. I have dealt with sensitive skin, an oily face, rosacea, and eczema since I was a child. I had a conversation with Ms. Hurley about her products. She was knowledgeable, understanding and encouraged me to try them. I was extremely reluctant to place oil on my face (placing oil on an oily face did not seem like a logical suggestion). Since I really had nothing to lose, I gave it a shot. I can't express how surprised I was when my face did not become oily and in fact the opposite occurred. My face has become very hydrated and balanced. My face is no longer oily!!! I have received numerous complements about how healthy my skin looks and how hydrated it feels. In addition, the oil has helped my crocodile elbows and heels, and has helped my rosacea and eczema. I use the oil every day after I shower and can immediately get dressed. It leaves no oily stains on my clothes and has no odor. I now use the facial cleaner, facial moisturizer, and lip balm as part of my daily routine. My husband now uses the lotion. Give it a try and you will be pleasantly surprised!

LISA ~ HASLET, TEXAS

Nourish has been so great for my son. When he was about a year old he started getting very large dry patches on his arms and thighs, along with red blotches on his face. He has always eaten very healthy, so we new it wasn't food related. We couldn't find anything that worked...until we started using Nourish! Within days, the dryness and red spots were gone and haven't returned since! So grateful we found these products!

LEE ~ PEORIA, AZ

I have been using Nourish Skin products now for several months as I came to you with very dry skin on my arms. I have tried several products but the two combinations of oil and cream products you suggested I use has been fantastic. My arms have literally cleared up and they stopped itching as well. Great job! I'll certainly recommend you and your great products!

SHERRIE ~ PEORIA, AZ

My skin is very dry and itchy. Have tried numerous products and nothing helped until I started using Nourish Body Lotion and Body Oil.

Within two days the itching stopped. I had no sensitivity to the products. Other products I have tried in the past caused hives and more itching. My skin has always been sensitive to products that have chemicals in them. The organic and botanical ingredients in Nourish Skin Care products are great for my skin. I am sure they will work for you, too.

KERRIE ~ DALLAS, TEXAS

Hello, as a makeup artist and licensed esthetician, I was really looking forward to trying your products. I am loving them so far and will be a customer. The ultra-moisturizing toner does exactly what it says it will, moisturizes your skin and gives you a pick me up. I also used it after swimming on my dry legs and it made them feel wonderful! I highly recommend these products!!

DARIS ~ FORT WORTH, TEXAS

I am an African American customer of the Nourish Skin Care Products. In the past I have been lead to believe that products are made for different skin types. I was very pleasantly surprised when I used the Nourish Skin Care Products to see how well they worked on my skin. I am particularly pleased on how smooth they make the skin feel and how light they are not leaving an oily residue. When my skin gets overly dry it gives an ashy appearance and with using the Nourish products I no longer have to worry about that as I always have a soft, hydrated and healthy look to my skin.

JANET ~ DES MOINES, IOWA

I was hesitant to use the Nourish oil on my face in the morning. Now I love, love, love it! Using the Nourish eye cream followed by the oil, morning and night, has replaced all of my other more expensive products and has streamlined my morning routine. My face feels much more healthy and smooth without all those products layered on under my makeup. I won't go back.

TONI ~ PHOENIX, AZ

I love the results that I have gotten from the Nourish product on the decollete area. I have sun-damaged skin in this area and the leathery look disappears when I apply the Nourish product.

CLEORA ~ PEORIA, AZ

I have been using the Nourish Your Skin Products for several weeks now and my skin is no longer itchy and dry. I no longer have cracked dry heels. I love your product.

FRAN ~ DENTON, TEXAS

I am 97 years old and live in Texas. I find the climate here very drying to my skin and I itch all of the time, I could hardly sleep at night for scratching my legs. I also had dry patches around my nose which looked terrible. I started using the Nourish product and the patches disappeared and I no longer itch. My skin doesn't feel like parchment paper anymore. Thank you Nourish.

SHERRIE, PEORIA, AZ

Nourish Organic Shampoo and Conditioner – I finally found a shampoo and conditioner that does not fade my color-treated hair – Nourish Organic Shampoo and Conditioner. I have been using the shampoo and conditioner for two months and my hair is healthy and has more volume. My hair is actually growing faster than ever before. I have received many compliments. My hairdresser said my hair is in wonderful condition. I will not use anything else! Highly recommend. Very pleasant fragrance.

MARY ANN Z. ~ PEORIA, AZ

I'm 54 years old and recently started getting facials regularly; my esthetician once said my skin is in better shape than hers is (she's late 20s, early 30s at most)! I guess after several visits she decided I must have done something to help my skin look so good; she finally asked if I had any "work" done or had Botox injections! I happily and proudly told her no, I've just been using "Nourish Your Skin" products for the last three years. Such great products; I'm proud to be a consultant for this company.

RITA ~ SUN CITY, AZ

How the oil helped my son – I want to tell you that I believe in miracles and giving my son the Nourish oil was a miracle. He was born with a birth defect that required his first surgery at 6 months. The doctor knew nothing about this problem, but found it necessary to operate on his arm. It took several surgeries and left his arm, from his fingers to his elbow, with skin that looked so bad. From the time he was little, he and I both bought and tried every kind of lotion that there was and never found anything that would keep that skin soft and from getting infections one after another. We visited with him in December and I left the bottle of oil and after the first night he told me he could not believe how good that arm felt. He said it is the first time he can remember seeing his arm nice and soft. Finally, after almost 57 years, he has found something to help him with this serious problem. Thank you! Thank you for this wonderful product. I just bought 2 more bottles of it and will be sending it to him.

CHRIS ~ PEORIA, AZ

I was born and raised in Arizona and was a sun worshiper. My skin was like a lizard. I tried every skin lotion imaginable from $10 to $100 per bottle and nothing worked until I tried the Nourish products. Within just a few days my skin felt soft and supple.

BARBARA ~ SUN CITY WEST, AZ

I use it daily to make my skin feel alive. Love it!

ANTOINETTE ~ PEORIA, AZ

Moving to Arizona caused my skin to become super sensitive, dry and I started having regular acne breakouts on my face. I have tried a variety of products that have caused immediate rash, irritation and redness. I am happy to say that I now use and LOVE the Nourish Lotion, Eye Creme and Facial Scrub. My skin looks great and I haven't had an acne breakout since.

SHERRY ~ PEORIA, AZ

I have never written about a product I use or even thought about doing so but there is one that I use every day that makes me feel good and puts a smile on my face - Nourish Ultra-Moisturing Toner. It is a perfect after-shower spray, smells great, feels better and I even like it more as I spritz my face after applying make-up. Sets my face with a moisturized feel and look all day. I won't even travel without it. Wonderful. 'Treat' your skin with this product.

KAYRA ~ SAGINAW, TEXAS

For the last two years, I have had the most enigmatic rashes all over my body. I slathered everything from coconut oil to raw Shea Butter to the finest of Essential Oils, and nothing helped. I knew if I went to a Dermatologist I would be given Prescriptions for Steroids in every form. Finally, my husband insisted I go to one that was supposed to take a more natural approach, but I left with a possible Lupus diagnosis, definite Fungus diagnosis on the face and neck, Dermatitis on the arms, Eczema Craquelle on the legs, and 5 different Steroidal Prescriptions. I tried the least dangerous-sounding ones, and promptly had a fierce escalation in symptoms. Plus, now I had a "Potentially Life Threatening Autoimmune Disease" diagnosis of Lupus hanging over my head! (Anyone with skin issues knows that stress can be the sole cause.)

I could use "over the counter" oils, creams and lotions and get things where I could function, but the swelling would not go down and never really clear up. Until I wore out all my old non-binding socks. I asked my Chiropractor if he knew where I could find natural fiber Diabetic socks. He gave me a Brochure for Linda Hurley's Nourish Skincare Products because she also has natural bamboo Diabetic-Friendly socks. On June 7, I left Linda's with 3 pr of Bamboo socks, a bottle of Nourish Skin Lotion and a bottle of Nourish Skin Oil.

June 20, I sent this email to Linda:

"All I can say is Praise the Eternal Almighty God for you and your products! My skin is almost all cleared up! Just a slight discoloration (scarring?) shows, but it is fading, too! My legs were swollen the day I spoke with you and now they are normal...I have lost two pounds of fluid! Does that tell you how swollen they were??"

I am so impressed that I have recommended these products to all my friends, especially to those with Dermatological issues.

DICTIONARY

ACRYLAMIDE (*uh*-kril-*uh*-mahyd) also known as olyacryl-amide. Used in facial moisturizers, anti-aging products, color cosmetics, lotions, hair products, sunscreens, and more. This chemical can affect you when breathe it in and by passing through your skin. Should be handled with care as a known carcinogen. Contact can cause eye irritation, watering, and inflammation.

ASTAXANTHIN (a-stə-ˈzan(t)-thən) Carotenoid (caro-tene pigment) is found in plants, algae, and fish, par-ticularly salmon, that functions as a potent antioxidant.

CAPILLARIES (kap-*uh*-ler-ee) Any one of the minute blood vessels between the terminations of the arteries and the beginnings of the veins.

COLLAGEN (kol-*uh*-juh n) This refers to any of a fam-ily of extracellular, closely related proteins occurring as a major component of connective tissue, giving it strength and flexibility.

DEHYDRATION (dee-hahy-**drey**-sh*uh* n) This occurs when you use or lose more fluid than you take in, and your body doesn't have enough water and other fluids to carry out its normal functions. If you don't replace lost fluids, you will get dehydrated.

DIHYDROXYACETONE (DHA) (dī'hī-drŏk'sē-ās'ĭ-tōn') This compound, also known as glycerone, is a simple carbohydrate with formula C3H6O3. DHA is primarily used as an ingredient in sunless tanning products. It is often derived from plant sources such as sugar beets and sugar cane, and by the fermentation of glycerin.

DIOXANE (dahy-ok-seyn) A flammable, potentially explosive, colorless liquid, $C_4H_8O_2$, that is used as a solvent for fats, greases, resins and in various products including paints, lacquers, glues, cosmetics, and fumigants.

FREE RADICALS (rad-i-*kuh* l z) Free radicals are unstable molecules that can damage the cells in your body. They form when atoms or molecules gain or lose electrons. They often occur as the result of normal metabolic processes. For example, when your body uses oxygen, it creates free radicals as a by-product and the damage caused by those free radicals is called 'oxidative stress.'

HYALURONIC ACID (hī(-ə) l-yu̇-'rä-nik) a glycosaminoglycan that is found in extra cellular tissue space, the synovial fluid of joints, and the vitreous humor of the eyes and acts as a binding, lubricating, and protective agent.

ISOPROPYL (SD-40) (ī-sə-prō-pəl) drying and irritating strips skin of natural acid mantle making skin vulnerable to bacteria, molds, and viruses.

MELANOCYTES (mə-la-nə-sīt) is a type of cell that's primarily located in the basal layer of the epidermis. Melanocytes produce melanin, a brown pigment that is responsible for skin coloration and protecting against the harmful effects of UV light. Melanocytes are also present in the hair and in the irises of the eyes.

MONOUNSATURATED FAT (mä-nō-ən-sa-chə-rā-təd) Monounsaturated fats are found in natural foods such as red meat, whole milk products, nuts and high fat fruits such as olives and avocados. Olive oil is about 75% mono-unsaturated fat

PARABENS (par-ə-benz) are synthetic preservatives used in foods, pharmaceuticals, cosmetics, and personal care products such as deodorants, moisturizers, and shampoos. Common parabens include methylparaben, ethylparaben, propylparaben and butylparaben. Parabens allow skin care products to survive for months or even years in your medicine cabinet; however, they also enter your body through your skin when you use these products. According to Mercola.com, the body can absorb as much as five pounds of cosmetic chemicals every year. Parabens can mimic hormones in the body and disrupt functions of the endocrine system.

PH - The pH scale measures how acidic or alkaline a substance is. The pH scale ranges from 0 to 14. A pH of 7 is neutral. A pH less than 7 is acidic. A pH greater than 7 is basic, or alkaline.

PHENOL CARBOLIC ACID (fē-nōl kär-bä-lik acid) a toxic white soluble crystalline acidic derivative of benzene; used in manufacturing and as a disinfectant and antiseptic; poisonous if taken internally

PROPYLENE GLYCOL (prō-pə-lēn glī-koٟl) a sweet, hygroscopic viscous liquid $C_3H_8O_2$ made especially from propylene and used especially as an antifreeze and solvent, in brake fluids, and as a food preservative

SODIUM LAURETH SULFATE (SLES) (sō-dē-əm lȯr-əth səl-fāt) is a concern as in some circumstances it can become contaminated with dioxane. This largely depends on the manufacturing process. Dioxane is a suspected carcinogen and lasts much longer in our bodies, primarily because the liver cannot metabolize it effectively. While it's considered less of a skin irritant when compared to SLS, there are underlying concerns over its continued use in beauty products.

SODIUM LAURYL SULFATE (SLS) (sō-dē-əm lȯr-əl səl-fāt) Sodium lauryl sulfate is a sulfate found in most shampoos that creates a great lather for cleansing, but is extremely harsh and drying. It is known to be one of the harshest surfactants due to its potential to be drying to the skin and hair.

SUN PROTECTION FACTOR (SPF) is simply a number on a scale for rating the degree of protection provided by sunscreens.

TOLUENE (täl-yə-wēn) is a colorless, liquid, flammable, poisonous hydrocarbon obtained originally from balsam of Tolu, but now generally from coal tar or petroleum, and used in making dyes, explosives, etc., and as a solvent

TRICLOSAN (trī-ˈklō-ˌsan) is an antibacterial agent and preservative used in personal care and home-cleaning products; persistent in the environment and may be associated with endocrine (hormonal) toxicity.

RESOURCES / REFERENCES

Lisa Henss - Director of Nutritional Counseling and Metabolic Testing. Clairton Family Chiropractic

Basic Biology of the Skin, Jones and Bartlett Learning

Organic Skin Care, Mary Beth Janssen

The Importance of Organic Skin Care, James Campbell

Toxic Ingredients in Cosmetics and Skin Care Products, Nicky Pilkington

United States Food and Drug Administration www.fda.com

Kids Health – www.kidshealth.org

WebMD – Men's Skincare – www.webmd.com

Active Beat, Lauren MacDonald

Melanoma Research Foundation (MRF)

International Agency for Research on Cancer (IARC)

Wow.com

ABOUT THE AUTHOR

Linda Irwin Hurley has been in the professional skin & hair care industry since the early 1960s. Starting her career as a hair stylist she quickly started opening her own chain of salons in southern California.

In the early 1970s, launching her company from the trunk of her car, she started her first distribution company, Joico West. Later she formed her corporation, Irwin Salon Services Inc., which distributed well-known professional hair and skin care products in the professional salon industry. Linda was fortunate to work with these companies from the ground floor, learning a lot about ingredients and formulations. Her company consisted of a large state-of-the-art facility with five satellite "Professional Only Stores" known as Professional West and a large outside sales force. In 2003, when the peak sales of her company had grown to $6 million dollars, she sold her company and retired to enjoy life.

In 2006, she relocated to Arizona. After enjoying retirement for three years and becoming increasingly disenchanted with too much idle time on her hands, she started thinking about ways to get active again. With the extreme dry climate in Arizona and with the downturn of the economy, she started looking around for something that could be beneficial to family, friends, and mankind in general. In 2009 Linda started working with a chemist, who assisted her in developing formulas for Nourish Your Skin Products.

Like many teenagers, Linda had an acne problem in her teens that left her forehead, cheeks and nose areas with extremely large pores and light scarring. Make-up covered the problem well but it was something that always bothered her. After using the Nourish Your Skin Product line for the past few years her pores have shrunk and the scarring has disappeared. Another benefit, her skin tone has completely evened out from its former mottled look, which gives her the option of wearing little or no makeup.

Recently Linda noticed a spot on her nose that obviously was caused by too much time in the sun as a teenager and she visited a skin cancer specialist who specializes in the Mohs Micrographic Surgery. Her doctor commented on the great texture and all around good health of her skin stating her skin has the appearance of a person 10 years younger than her chronological years. All thanks to following the skin care regimen outlined in this book.

Linda currently lives in Fort Worth, Texas.

If you would like more information on the "Nourish Your Skin" products or would like to place an order please visit our website:

www.nourishskincareproducts.com

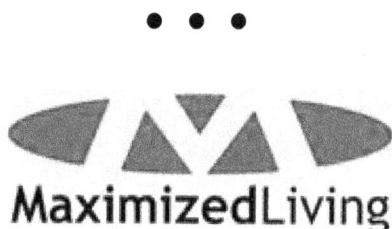

• • •

MaximizedLiving

Dr. Bryan Henss
Clairton Family Chiropractic
A Maximized Living Health Center
8333 Sohi Dr, Ste 102, Fort Worth, TX 76137
817.281.1400
www.clairtonfamilychiro.com

DR. BRYAN HENSS IS A leader in a global network of doc-
tors at the forefront of healthcare. He serves on the USA
Sports Performance Council for various Olympic teams.
He has received advanced certifications in spinal correc-
tion, nutrition, fitness, pediatrics, and pregnancy care. In
addition to running a rapidly growing health center lo-
cally, Dr. Bryan's heart is for serving people throughout
the community. He donates his time to help churches

incorporate comprehensive wellness programs, teaching them God's laws of health and healing. He has delivered these programs to corporations, schools, sports teams, and organizations as well.

After watching his mother lose her health, he found his passion for Chiropractic during his studies in kinesiology at Illinois College, which prompted him to ask the tough questions about health and how the human body works. While exploring options in healthcare, the principles of Maximized Living stood out from the rest: to find the cause of health problems, remove the interference, and maximize potential.

Dr. Bryan attended Logan College of Chiropractic in St. Louis, MO. Since then he has had the privilege of working alongside some of the most distinguished and renowned chiropractors in North America, including training in the largest pediatric practice in the Midwest. Dr. Bryan is a husband to Lisa and father to their son Lane. He enjoys golfing, baseball, football, and spending time with his family.